The Skinny 5:2 Diet Family Favourites Recipe Book

Eat With All The Family On Your Diet Fasting Days.

Skinny 5:2 Recipe Ideas For All The Family To Enjoy Under 300, 400 And 500 Calories

D1374993

CookNation

Copyright

ISBN-13: 978-1483941424

Disclaimer

The information and advice in this book is intended as a guide only. Any individual should independently seek the advice of a health professional before embarking on a diet.

Contents

Contents (cont)

Introduction

Are you following the 5:2 Fast Diet plan but also have a family to prepare meals for every day?

Following the 5:2 Fast Diet while still looking after your family can be a tricky balance. Planning your own low calorie meals for your fasting days whilst thinking what to cook for everyone else can be an extra pressure you don't need and makes sticking to your diet plan all the more difficult.

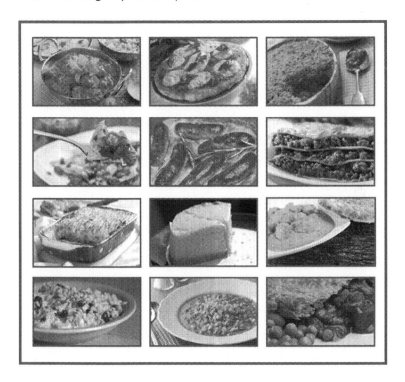

It doesn't have to be that way.

In the Skinny 5:2 Fast Diet Family Favourites Recipe Book

we've selected some all-time favourite family meals that you can all enjoy and eat together, safe in the knowledge that you are keeping to your fast day calorie limit, but still providing for your family.

The dishes are all classic meals, snacks and desserts which your family will love and they are easy to prepare. What's more, each skinny recipe falls under either 300, 400 or 500 calories making your 5:2 efforts ...effortless.

We hope that you and your family enjoy these recipes and good luck with your 5:2 plan!

About The 5:2 Diet

Imagine a diet where you can eat whatever you want for 5 days a week and fast for 2. That's what the 5:2 Diet is and it's revolutionised the way people think about dieting.

By allowing you the freedom to eat normally for MOST of the week and restrict your calorie intake for just TWO non-consecutive days a week (500 calories per day for women and 600 for men) you keep yourself motivated and remove that dreaded feeling of constantly denying yourself the food you really want to eat.

It still takes willpower but it's nowhere near as much of a grind when you know you've got tomorrow to look forward to. It's all about freedom. You choose when and you choose what you want to eat and with 'The Skinny 5:2 Diet Family Favourites Recipe Book' balancing your family's meals couldn't be easier.

Popularised by Dr. Michael J. Mosley the 5:2 diet plan has been adopted by both health professionals and regular people alike as a way of life which will change your relationship with dieting and weight loss. What's more this way of eating is believed to have major well-being benefits which could alter your health forever.

How It Works

The concept of fasting is an ancient one and modern science is uncovering evidence that fasting can be an extremely healthy way to shed extra weight. Research has shown that it can reduce levels of IGF-1 (insulin-like growth factor 1, which leads to accelerated ageing), activate DNA repair genes and reduce blood pressure, cholesterol and glucose levels.

This book has been developed specifically to help you concentrate on the practice of 5:2, if you want to find out more about the specific details of the science of the subject we would recommend Dr. Michael J. Mosley's work and, as with all diets, you should consider seeking advice from a health professional before starting.

Taking It Week By Week

The 5:2 Diet can work for you whatever your lifestyle. Each week you should think carefully about which days are likely to be best suited to your fasting days and then stick with it. You can change your days each week or keep in a regular routine, whichever suits you best as long as your fasting days are non-consecutive.

Of course, reducing your calorie intake for two days will take some getting used to and inevitably there will be hunger pangs to start with, but you'll be amazed at how quickly your body adapts to your new style of eating and far from gorging the day after your fasting day you'll find you simply enjoy the luxury of eating normally.

The Family Favourite recipes in this book have been designed to fill you up as much as possible during your fasting days. Most recipes serve 4, so if you are cooking only for yourself you can freeze into meal size portions for easy use over the coming weeks.

Some 5:2 Tips

Avoid too much exercise on your fasting days. Eating less is likely to make you feel a little weaker, certainly to start with, so don't put the pressure on yourself to exercise.

Avoid alcohol on your fasting days. Not only is alcohol packed with calories, it could also have a greater effect on you than usual as you haven't eaten as much.

Don't give up! Even if you find your fasting days tough to start with, stick with it. Remember you can eat what you like tomorrow without having to feel guilty.

Remember it's you that's dieting not your family!

It's important to remember that while each of the recipes in this book are within the daily calorific limit of the 5:2 diet plan and can be enjoyed by everyone, don't forget that the rest of your family may not be following a diet. Therefore, it's equally important that they meet their own daily calorie intakes through other meals and snacks. The recommend daily calorie intakes are as follows:

Age	Boys	Girls
1–3	1,230	1,165
4–6	1,715	1,545
7–10	1,970	1,740
11–14	2,220	1,845
15–18	2,755	2,110
Adults	2,550	1,940

If you are pregnant, breastfeeding, diabetic or suffer form any health issues, you should consult a health professional before embarking on any diet plan.

Nutrition

All of the recipes in this collection are balanced low calorie family meals which should keep you feeling full on your fasting days. All recipes have serving suggestions; the calories noted on the recipes are per serving of the recipe ingredients only, so bear that in mind.

Please give us your feedback

We'd love to hear about your 5:2 diet experiences so feel

free to leave a review. Reviews help others decide if this is the right book for them so a moment of your time would be very welcome. Thank you.

CookNation

Meals

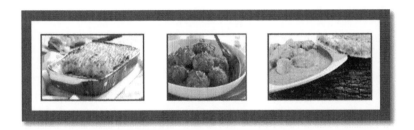

BBQ Pulled Pork

Serves 5-6

Calories per serving: 262

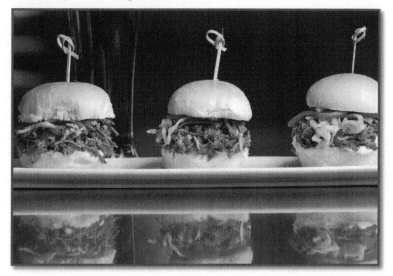

Pulled pork is an absolute classic. It's a chance to use just about everything in your spice rack to create a killer dry rub and it always packs an irresistible punchy and more-ish taste.

Ingredients:

1.8kg pork butt (shoulder)

1 onion, chopped

250ml BBQ sauce or ketchup

500ml beef stock or boiling water

1 packet BBQ dry rub

Or make your own...

1 tbsp each of garlic powder, brown sugar, onion powder,

celery salt, paprika, chili powder & cumin

Method:

Preheat the oven to 275F/140C/Gas Mark 1

Combine all the spices together and cover the pork in the dry spice rub. Add the stock, onion & BBQ sauce to a roasting tin and then place the pork on top. Cover the tin really tightly with foil and leave to cook for aprox 5-6 hrs. Ideally you should turn the pork half way through cooking but if you can't don't worry too much. Measure the internal temperature of the meat. The pork will be cooked at around 160°, but won't fall apart perfectly until 190°. Leave to rest for as long as you can resist and then use your hands or 2 forks to pull the pork apart. Once it's all shredded, place in a bowl and remove the cooking liquid from the slow cooker. Pour the liquid onto the pork to make beautiful juicy meat that you can enjoy with just about everything - whether it's a light salad or sandwich rolls with hot sauce and salad.

Beef Stew

Serves: 4

Calories per serving: 371

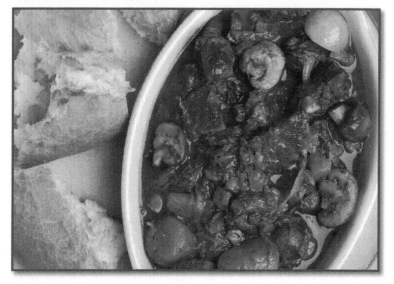

Beef stew is a national institution. Use the best stewing steak you can to get the most out of the stew and don't worry if you don't have red wine, just increase the stock quantities.

Ingredients:

600g stewing beef, trimmed and cubed

1 tbsp plain flour

100g lean back bacon

1 tbsp Worcestershire sauce

1 onion, chopped

2 carrots, chopped

4 cloves garlic, crushed

50g mushrooms, sliced

1 tsp each chopped thyme & oregano

300ml red wine

500ml beef stock

Low cal cooking spray

Salt & pepper to taste

Method:

Preheat the oven to 300F/150C/Gas Mark 2

Brown the beef in a frying pan with a little low cal cooking spray. Remove the beef and place in a plastic bag with the flour and shake well to cover the meat. Meanwhile cook the bacon in the same frying pan. Add the onions, garlic, carrots and mushrooms and leave to cook gently. Season well. Add the contents of your pan plus the beef into a casserole dish and pour in the wine and stock before bringing to the boil on the hob. Cover and place in the oven for 2-3 hrs or until the meat is really tender. The flour on the beef should ensure the stew is thick enough, but if not you can reduce the liquid by cooking on a high heat over the hob with the lid off for a few minutes longer.

Biryani

Serves: 4
Calories per serving: 461

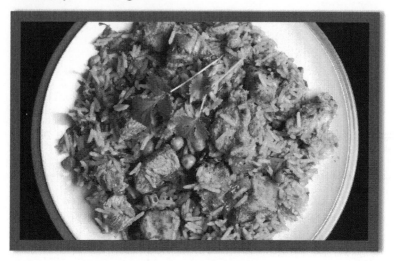

This version of the classic spiced rice and sauce dish prepares both elements separately before combining right at the end.

Curry Ingredients:

300g lean meat diced
4 portions *skinny curry base mix* **(see page 70 for recipe)**
2 tsp mild curry powder
½ tsp salt
1 tsp sugar
3 tbsp tomato puree
85g frozen peas
½ tsp each ground garlic, cumin, coriander, paprika & turmeric powder
100ml single cream
1 tsp sunflower oil

Rice Ingredients:

200g basmati rice
½ onion, finely chopped
¼ tsp ground cinnamon
¼ tsp ground cloves
1 bay leaf
Pinch of Saffron
1 chicken stock cube
1 tsp sunflower oil
Salt & pepper to taste

Method:
Brown the meat in a frying pan with the sunflower oil. Add the dried spices, curry powder and tomato puree and gently cook for a minute or two. Add the skinny curry base mix, peas, sugar & salt and leave to cook for 20 minutes or until the meat is tender and completely cooked through.

Boil a pan of water and dissolve a cube of chicken stock into it. Meanwhile, gently fry the onion, cinnamon and cloves for a few minutes in the sunflower oil. Add the rice to the pan and coat well with the oil. Transfer contents of frying pan plus the bay leaf and saffron into the boiling stock water and cook until tender.

When both the rice and curry are ready take off the heat and stir the cream through. Combine the rice and curry together to make a takeaway style biryani.

Cheese Steak Sandwich

Serves: 4

Calories per serving: 445

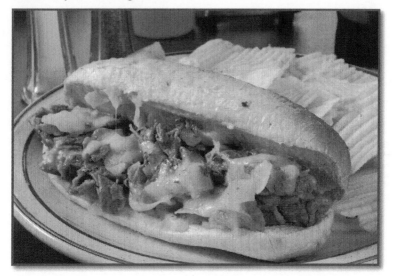

A cheese steak sandwich is the ultimate wholesome fast food. Make sure your cheese is melted before digging in.

Ingredients:

450g lean flank or skirt steak, trimmed

1 onion, sliced

50g mushrooms, sliced

1 red pepper, chopped

2 tsp Worcestershire sauce

4 low fat cheese slices

1 tbsp fresh oregano

Salt & pepper to taste

Low cal cooking spray

4 low fat sandwich rolls

Method:

Preheat oven to 375°F/190C/Gas Mark 5
Gently fry the onion, pepper and mushrooms in a frying pan
with some low calorie cooking spray. When they are soft add
the oregano and Worcestershire sauce and cook for a minute
longer. Remove to a plate and turn up the heat. Season and fry
the steak for a couple of minutes each side (or longer for well
done). Allow the steak to rest for a few minutes and then slice
as thinly as possible.
Divide the meat and onion mixture across the sandwich rolls
and place a cheese slice on top. Close the sandwich roll over
and individually wrap in foil. Place in the preheated oven for 5-
10 mins.

Chicken Goujons

Serves: 4

Calories per serving: 338

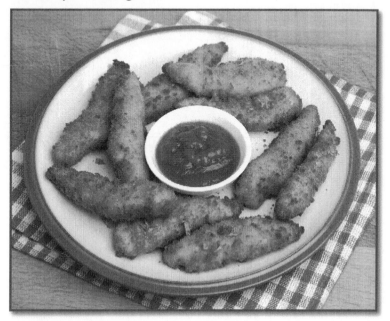

Homemade chicken goujons are a healthy alternative to the universally loved chicken nugget... and the good news is the kids should enjoy them just as much!

Ingredients:

3 slices white bread

1 clove garlic

30g grated parmesan cheese

500g skinless chicken breasts, cut into strips

50g plain flour

2 free range eggs

Low cal cooking spray

Salt & pepper to taste

Method:

Preheat the oven to 190C/375F/Gas Mark 5.

First make the breadcrumbs. Put the bread, garlic, cheese and a pinch of salt and pepper into a food processor and whizz until you have breadcrumbs.

Put the flour onto a plate, the breadcrumbs on a separate plate and beat the eggs in a bowl. Cover each chicken strip with flour by rolling them on the flour plate and then dip each strip in the egg. Finally, coat well in breadcrumbs.

Place on a grilling rack on top of a baking tray and leave to cook for 15 minutes or until golden brown and cooked through. Serve with lemon wedges, ketchup, salad and sandwich rolls.

Chicken Risotto

Serves: 4

Calories Per Serving: 430

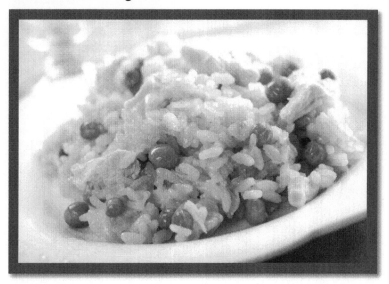

Usually served as a first course in Italy, this roast chicken version makes a beautiful main meal.

Ingredients:

1 tbsp olive oil

Knob butter

1 large onion, chopped

2 garlic cloves, chopped

225g risotto rice

1lt vegetable stock

225g left over roast chicken, chopped

100g peas

Method:

Sauté the onion and garlic in the oil and butter for a few minutes. Add the risotto rice to the pan and make sure each grain is coated well with the oil and butter. Gradually add the stock a ladle at a time, stirring until the liquid is absorbed each time before adding the next ladle. After 10 mins of cooking add the peas.

Make sure the risotto is tender and add the roast chicken to warm through for a few minutes. Serve with a basil garnish and plain rocket salad with parmesan cheese shavings.

Chilli Con Carne

Serves: 4

Calories per serving: 440

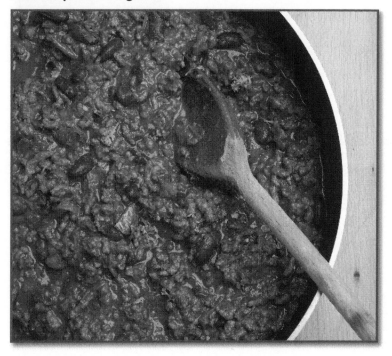

The Spanish name simply means 'chilli with meat' and this dish has been a Tex-Mex classic since before the days of the American frontier settlers. Slow cooking the mince beef really allows the flavour to develop.

Ingredients:

500g lean minced beef

1 400g tin chopped tomatoes

1 400g tin kidney beans, drained

1 large onion chopped

1 beef stock cube dissolved into 250ml water

500g tomato passata

1 tsp each brown sugar, oregano, cumin, mild chilli powder, paprika & garlic

½ tsp salt

Low cal cooking spray

Method:

Brown the mince and onions in a frying pan with a little low cal spray. Combine all the ingredients into a sauce pan, bring up to heat, cover and leave to cook on low for 60 minutes. Ensure the meat is fully cooked through and serve with rice or tortilla chips and a dollop of fat free Greek yoghurt. For a fuller flavour leave to cook for longer on a lower heat.

Corned Beef Hash

Serves: 4

Calories per serving: 431

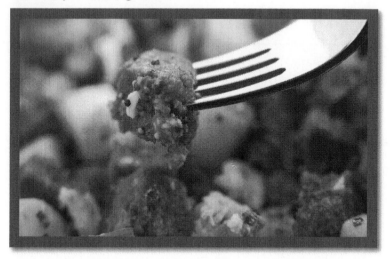

Corned beef hash is very simple to make. We don't tend to make corned beef from scratch in the UK so it's fine to use tinned.

Ingredients:

500g lean corned beef

500g potatoes, peeled and cubed

100g chopped cabbage

1 large onion, sliced

Pinch crushed chilli flakes

200ml beef stock

Low cal cooking spray

Salt & pepper to taste

Method:

Spray a pan with a little low-cal cooking spray and gently fry the onions for a few minutes. Add the potatoes, cabbage, chilli flakes, corned beef and stock, cover and leave to cook gently for approx 30 mins. When the liquid has been absorbed and the potatoes are tender remove from the pan and serve.

Cowboy Casserole

Serves: 4

Calories per serving: 414

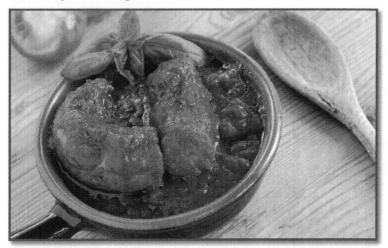

Loved by kids and adults alike this is a real cowboy's suppertime meal which always goes down a treat. It takes just minutes to put together and is a great way to get some veggies into the kids.

Ingredients:

8 lean pork sausages

2 400g tins mixed beans, drained

2 400g tins chopped tomatoes

1 onion, chopped

2 carrots, chopped

1 tbsp tomato puree or ketchup

1 tsp brown sugar

1 tsp dijon mustard

50ml vegetable stock or boiling water

Low cal cooking spray

Method:

Brown the sausages in the pan with the onions and a little low cal cooking spray. Cut the sausages into bite-size slices and combine with all the other ingredients in an uncovered saucepan and leave to cook gently for 60 mins. Check the sausages are properly cooked and serve with crusty bread or mashed potato and green vegetables.

Fajitas

Serves: 4

Calories per serving: 270

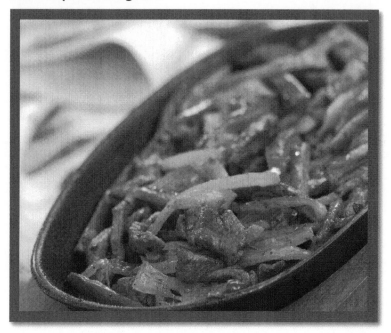

Steak is the Fajita meat of choice. Make sure you trim the meat as much as possible to give you a lean cut. Slice as thinly as you can when cooked.

Ingredients:

400g steak

1 large onion, sliced

3 peppers, deseeded and sliced (any colour is fine)

2 tbsp lime juice

Steak spice mix:

1 tsp mild chilli powder, ½ tsp ground cumin, ½ tsp paprika, ¼ tsp each of onion powder, garlic powder, dried oregano & crushed chilli flakes

Salt & pepper to taste

Low-cal cooking spray

Method:

Combine the steak spice mix and lime juice together and brush all over the steak. Cover and leave to chill for an hour or two if possible.

Spray a frying pan with a little low-cal cooking oil and get the pan nice and hot. Add the steak and cook for 3-4 minutes each side (for medium) or longer/less if you prefer. Remove from the pan, cover in foil and leave to rest. Meanwhile, use the same pan to gently cook the onions and peppers until tender. When they are softened uncover the steak and slice as thinly as possible and mix with the onions and peppers.

Serve with low-cal flour tortillas, grated cheese, salsa, salad & sour cream.

Family Pizza

Serves: 4

Calories per serving: 460

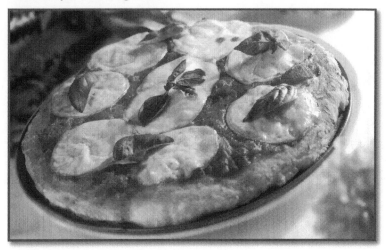

This simple pizza can be altered to suit your family's taste. Experiment with toppings but watch the calories on any additional ingredients.

Ingredients:

1 packet yeast
125g whole-wheat flour
125g all-purpose flour
2 tsp runny honey
½ salt
¾ tbsp extra-virgin olive oil
180ml warm water

Toppings:

4 tbsp tomato puree
2 tsp garlic paste
200g low fat mozzarella cheese, cubed
2 tbsp parmesan cheese, freshly grated
Salt and pepper to taste
Fresh basil
Drizzle olive oil

Method:

Preheat the oven to 425F/220C/Gas Mark 7

Place the yeast, warm water and honey in a mixer and leave to stand for a minute or two. Start the mixer and slowly add the flour. When everything starts to combine add the olive oil and salt. Carefully mix until it becomes a dough. As soon as the dough is formed take out of the mixer and bring together into one ball.

Leave to rest for about half an hour or until the dough has increased to approx. double its original size. Cut the dough in two and roll into two 25-30cm pizzas. It's best to roll out onto a piece of baking parchment so that you can put straight onto a baking tray.

Mix the tomato and garlic purees together and spread out the puree mix onto the dough discs to make a base on each. Arrange the cubed mozzarella evenly over the two dough discs and a drizzle a little olive oil on top.

Leave to cook in the oven for about 8-10 minutes, or until the base is properly cooked. Remove from the oven and sprinkle with fresh parmesan and basil.

Finger Licking Rack Of Ribs

Serves: 5
Calories per serving: 448

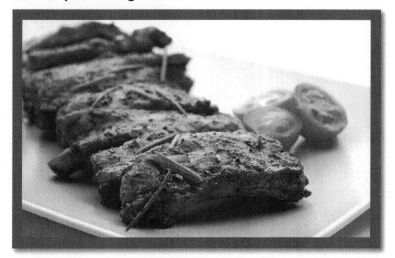

There are a number of different types of ribs available depending on the cut from which they are taken. Choose whichever is cheapest or whichever you prefer. All will work well with this recipe.

Ingredients:

1.1kg pork ribs

1 tsp each garlic powder, chilli, cumin & basil

½ tsp salt

2 400g tins chopped tomatoes

1 tbsp ketchup

1 red chilli, chopped or a pinch crushed chilli flakes to taste

Method:

Preheat the oven to 325F/170C/Gas Mark 3

Rub the dry spices onto the ribs. Add all the ingredients to a roasting tin making sure the tomatoes cover the ribs. Cover tightly with foil and leave to cook for 2-2 ½ hours. Ensure the ribs are cooked through and tender before serving with rice and beans.

Fish & Chips

Serves: 4
Calories per serving: 486

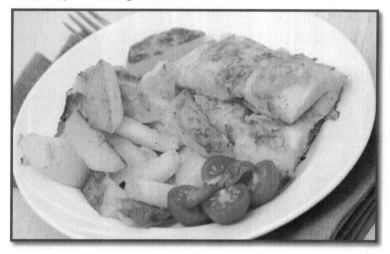

Here's a low calorie alternative to the usual deep fried fish and chips. Choose whichever white fish you prefer, or whatever is on offer at the supermarket.

Ingredients:

400g desiree potatoes, skin on

Low calorie cooking spray

1 tsp crushed sea salt

2 tbsp plain flour

3 slices white bread

20g grated parmesan cheese

1 garlic clove

2 free range eggs

700g meaty white fish fillets (haddock or pollack)

Method:

Preheat oven to 200C/400F/Gas6

Cut the potatoes into 'chips'. These should be about 2cm wide. Put in a bowl and spray well with low cal cooking oil. Make sure every chip is covered and add the salt. Mix well. Place on a baking tray and cook in the oven for approx. 25-30 minutes or until golden brown, crispy and tender. Increase the temperature for the last part of cooking if necessary.

Meanwhile make the breadcrumbs by putting the bread, garlic, cheese and a pinch of salt and pepper into a food processor and whizzing until you have breadcrumbs.

Put the flour onto a plate, the breadcrumbs on a separate plate and beat the eggs in a bowl. Cover each fish fillet with flour by turning them on the flour plate and then dip each fillet in the egg. Finally coat well in the breadcrumbs.

Put to one side and place a frying pan on a medium to high heat with some low calorie cooking spray. Carefully fry the fish for 2-3 minutes on each side or until golden and cooked through. Serve with lemon wedges and cherry tomatoes or mushy peas!

Fish Pie

Serves: 4

Calories per serving: 470

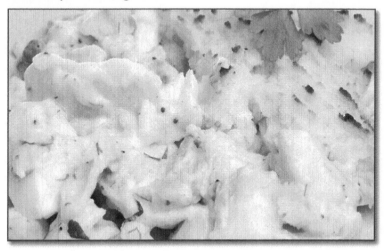

Fish pie is pure comfort food. The version here is very simple to suit the kids' palette but you'll enjoy it too! You could add prawns and salmon to this to increase colour and flavour.

Ingredients:

225g smoked haddock fillets

225g haddock fillets (or whichever white fish you prefer)

800g desiree potatoes, peeled and cubed

100g frozen peas

100g frozen sweet corn

1 large carrot, finely chopped

100g low fat cheddar cheese, grated

40g low fat 'butter' spread

750ml skimmed milk

1 tsp Dijon mustard (or less if that doesn't suit everyone)

Method:

Preheat the oven to 200C/400F/Gas Mark 6

Place the fish in a pan and cover with milk (you won't need to use all the milk here). Gently poach for a few minutes until the fish breaks apart when you try to separate it. Remove the fish from the pan and keep the milk.

Cook the sweetcorn, carrots & peas and when tender place in an oven proof dish with the cooked fish.

Meanwhile, cook the potatoes in salted boiling water until tender. When they are ready, drain and mash using half the butter and a splash of the fishy milk.

Gently melt the other 20g of butter in a pan and stir through the flour. When you have a nice paste begin adding all the milk gradually (including the fishy milk). The sauce will thicken after a minute or two. Add the mustard and cheese, remove from the heat and pour onto the fish and vegetables.

Cover with the smooth mash and cook for approx. 25-30 minutes or until golden brown and cooked through.

Homemade Cheese Burger

Serves: 4

Calories per serving: 345

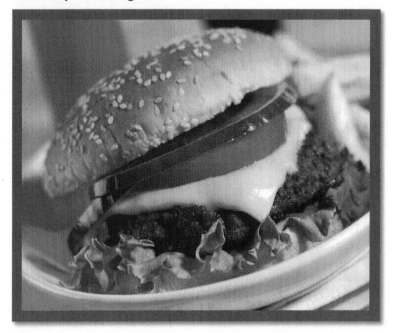

Everyone loves a good burger and making them yourself at home ensures you know exactly what goes into them.

Ingredients:

280g lean minced beef

50g breadcrumbs

50g carrots, grated

1 onion, grated

1 tsp Worcestershire sauce

4 low fat cheese slices

½ Romaine lettuce shredded

2 tomatoes, sliced

4 low calorie burger buns

Salt & pepper to taste

Method:

Mix all the ingredients, except the cheese, salad and burger buns, together. When the mixture is well combined use a burger shaper, or your hands, to make 4 meat patties.

Grill the burgers for approx. 8 mins, then place a cheese slice on top of each burger and grill for a further 2 minutes or until the burgers are cooked through. Place a burger in each bun with the tomatoes and lettuce.

Italian Meatballs

Serves: 4

Calories per serving: 323

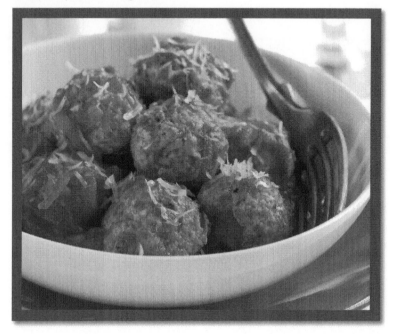

Meatballs are easy to make and never a disappointment to eat. The simple sauce accompanying the meat here is lovely as it is, but a dash of Worcestershire sauce or a tsp of marmite will give it additional depth.

Ingredients:

500g lean ground beef

1 slice of bread whizzed into bread crumbs

½ onion, finely chopped

Handful fresh parsley chopped

1 free range egg

1 clove garlic, crushed

1 tsp salt

2 400g tins chopped tomatoes

2 tbsp tomato puree

250ml beef stock

1 tsp each of dried basil, oregano & thyme

Method:

Preheat the oven to 350F/180C/Gas Mark 4.

Combine together the beef, breadcrumbs, egg, onion, garlic and half the salt. (You can do it with your hands or for super-speed put it all into a food mixer).

Once the ingredients are properly mixed together use your hands to shape into about 20-24 meatballs and place in the pre heated oven for 20-25 mins or until cooked through.

Meanwhile, add all the other ingredients to a pan and heat gently while the meatballs cook. When they are ready transfer into the pan. Cover and leave to simmer for a few minutes. Serve with spaghetti, parmesan and a green salad.

Jambalaya

Serves: 4

Calories per serving: 320

Seafood, meat and rice are the basis for Jambalaya. For a more southern taste, leave out the chopped tomatoes and increase the Cajun seasoning.

Ingredients:

175g skinless chicken breasts, cubed

175g king prawns, chopped

1 onion, diced

1 red pepper, thinly sliced

2 garlic cloves, crushed

1 stalk celery, chopped

50g chorizo sausage, diced

200g long grain rice

1 400g tin chopped tomatoes

250ml chicken stock

3 spring onions, chopped

Low cal cooking spray

1 tbsp cajun seasoning

Or make your own:

1 tsp paprika

1 tsp salt

1/2 tsp garlic powder

1 tsp crushed chillies

1 tsp dried oregano

½ tsp ground coriander

Method:

Spray a frying pan with a little low-cal cooking spray and brown the chicken for a few minutes on a high heat. Remove the meat and gently fry the onions for a few minutes before adding the peppers, celery, garlic, sausage, prawns and cajun seasoning. Leave to cook for a few minutes then add the chicken, rice, chopped tomatoes and stock. Cover and simmer for 20-25 mins until the rice is tender and the liquid is absorbed.

Kedgeree

Serves: 4

Calories per serving: 444

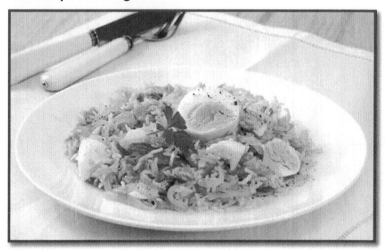

This rice and fish dish is thought to have originated in India making it's way back to the UK as part of the Empire's connections. Kedgeree can be eaten hot or cold and you can substitute other fish such as tuna or salmon, if you prefer.

Ingredients:

1 tsp low fat 'butter' spread

1 onion, chopped

¼ tsp turmeric

¼ tsp ground cinnamon

1 bay leaf

450g basmati rice

1 litre chicken stock

750g smoked haddock skinless, boneless fillets

3 free range eggs

1 lemon

Salt & pepper to taste

Method:

Melt the butter spread in a saucepan and gently cook the onions for a few minutes. Add the rice and spices and coat well in the butter and onions. Add the stock and bay leaf, season well, cover and leave to cook for 10 minutes. Meanwhile, hard boil the eggs, peel and cut into quarters lengthwise, and in a shallow pan gently poach the fish in water until the flesh flakes (about 5 mins). Remove the fish to a plate and flake. Check the rice is tender and all the stock is absorbed. Take out the bay leaf and gently combine with the fish and eggs. Serve in bowls with a wedge of lemon each.

Korma

Serves 4

Calories per serving 359

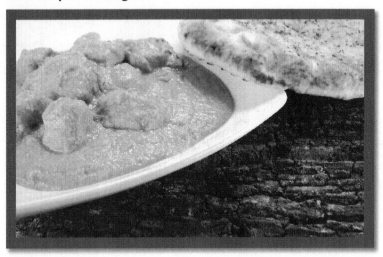

A mild, yellow curry, Korma always contains almonds and/or coconut. This skinny version uses low fat coconut milk.

Ingredients:

2 portions skinny curry base mix **(see page 70 for recipe)**

600g lean meat cubed

1 tsp mild curry powder

¼ tsp ground ginger

½ tsp ground garlic, turmeric, garam masala, cumin

1 bay leaf

100ml low fat coconut milk

1 tsp sugar

½ tsp salt

Few drops natural yellow food colouring

2 tsp sunflower oil

Method:

Add the sunflower oil to a frying pan and brown your meat on a medium/high heat. Meanwhile, mix the dry spices in a cup with a little water to make a smooth paste. Turn the meat to a low heat, add the spice paste, sugar, bay leaf and skinny curry base mix. Stir well and leave to simmer for approx. 20 minutes or until the meat is properly cooked through.

Finally, add the coconut milk and food colouring, warm through gently and serve.

Lancashire Hotpot

Serves: 4

Calories per serving: 474

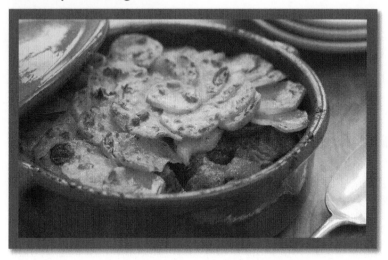

Hotpot is traditionally made from lamb or mutton and onion and topped with sliced potatoes. It is often served at large family gatherings as it is so easy to prepare and doesn't cost a lot. The ingredients here serve 4 - you can easily double up to feed more.

Ingredients:

500g lean lamb, cut into large chunks

2 onions, chopped

4 carrots, sliced

25g plain flour

1 tbsp Worcestershire sauce

500ml lamb stock

1 bay leaf

1 tsp dried thyme

400g potatoes, peeled and thinly sliced

Low calorie cooking spray

Salt & pepper to taste

Method:

Preheat the oven to 325F/170C/Gas Mark 3.

In an oven proof dish brown the lamb with some low cal cooking spray. Put to one side and gently fry the carrots and onion in the same dish for a few minutes using a little more low cal spray if needed. Add the flour and stir well, pour in the stock and Worcestershire sauce and bring to the boil. Take off the heat, add the meat and stir. Arrange the potato slices over the top, spray cooking oil and place in the preheated oven for 2 hours or until the meat is cooked and the potatoes tender. You can leave it in for longer on a lower heat, and if you want it browned off put under a hot grill for a couple of minutes.

Lasagne

Serves: 6

Calories per serving: 420

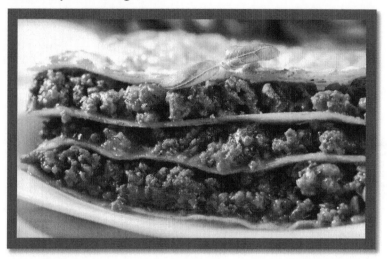

This is a big lasagne which will last a couple of meals for a smaller family. Bulk up with a fresh green salad when serving.

Ingredients:

1 onion, chopped

3 garlic cloves, crushed

1 400g tin chopped tomatoes

1 tbsp worcestershire sauce

½ tsp salt

250ml tomato passata

500g lean minced turkey

100g low fat ricotta cheese

50g low fat mozzarella cheese, cubed

50g low fat cheddar, grated

1 free range egg, beaten

150g lasagne sheets

Low cal cooking spray

Method:

Preheat the oven to 375F/190C/Gas Mark 5

Fry the turkey, onion and garlic in the low cal oil for 5 mins. Add the chopped tomatoes, puree, salt and Worcestershire sauce and cook for a further 10 minutes. Meanwhile mix the ricotta, mozzarella and eggs together. In a baking dish, layer the lasagne sheets, meat and cheese mixes, finishing with a layer of meat on which the grated cheddar is sprinkled.

Cover and cook for 45 minutes. Remove the foil and bake for a further 10-15 to brown off the cheese. Ensure the lasagne is properly cooked through and serve.

Macaroni Cheese

Serves: 4

Calories Per Serving: 380

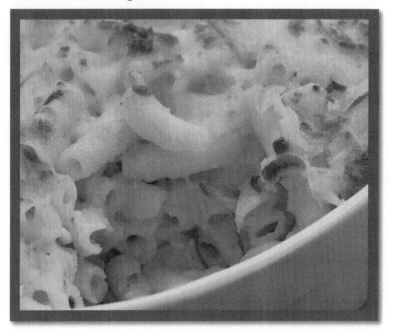

Using the evaporated milk in this recipe makes for a lovely creamy consistency. Make sure you don't overcook the macaroni.

Ingredients:

225g macaroni pasta

200g low fat cheddar cheese, grated

1 tsp dijon mustard

100ml evaporated milk

400ml skimmed milk

2 free range eggs, beaten

Knob of butter

½ tsp nutmeg

Method:

Preheat the oven to 350F/180C/Gas Mark 4

Cook the macaroni pasta until al dente. Meanwhile, gently combine all the other ingredients (except the nutmeg) in a bowl and when the pasta is ready, drain and add this to your mixture. Mix well and pour everything into an ovenproof dish and place in the pre heated oven for 30 minutes or until piping hot. Sprinkle with nutmeg before serving.

Marmite Spaghetti

Serves 4:

Calories per serving:198

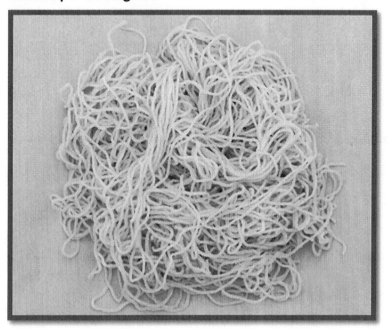

Love it or hate it Marmite is just about as British as it gets! Marmite Spaghetti may seem an unusual combination but it was popularised by Italian food writer Anna Del Conte and has become a modern student classic. The saltiness of the marmite and the silkiness of the butter on spaghetti make for a winning combination.

Ingredients:

300g spaghetti or linguine

25g unsalted butter

1 heaped tsp marmite (or more to taste)

Salt & pepper to taste

30g grated parmesan

Squirt of ketchup

Method:

Bring a pan of salted water to the boil and cook the spaghetti until tender.

While the pasta is cooking gently heat together the marmite and butter in a large saucepan. When the spaghetti is ready, reserve a ladle of the pasta water before draining. Add the drained spaghetti to the marmite pan and mix well to make sure every strand is covered with the buttery marmite mix.

If the spaghetti is a little sticky, add a splash of the reserved pasta water to loosen it up and divide into bowls. Use squeezy ketchup to make a swirl on the top of the spaghetti and sprinkle with parmesan. Surprisingly delicious!

Nachos

Serves: 4

Calories per serving: 324

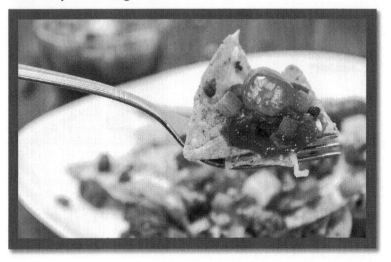

Inspired by the flavours of Tex Mex this dish is great fun to eat as a family with everyone helping themselves across the table.

Ingredients:

500g lean minced beef

1 onion, chopped

1 pepper, chopped

200g low fat refried beans

2 400g tins chopped tomatoes

150ml beef stock

Chilli to taste!

4 tsp taco seasoning

Or make your own:

2 tsp mild chilli powder, 1 ½ tsp ground cumin, ½ tsp paprika, onion powder, garlic powder & dried oregano, 1 tsp each of sea salt & black pepper

Method:

Brown the mince and onions in a frying pan. Add the taco seasoning and continue to cook for a minute or two. Combine all the ingredients into a saucepan, bring up to heat, cover and leave to cook on low for approx. 60 minutes. Ensure the beef is well cooked and serve with tortilla chips, shredded salad, grated cheese, guacamole and sour cream (or fat free Greek yoghurt).

Omelette

Serves: 1

Calories per serving: 330

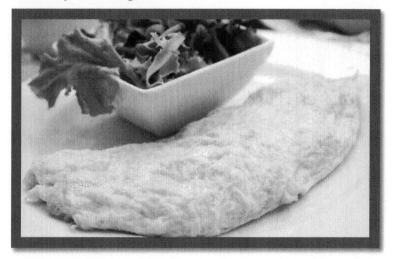

This recipe is for a single large omelette. You can make them one by one and keep warm in the oven or have a couple of pans going at the same time.

Ingredients:

3 free range eggs, beaten

¼ red onion, chopped

½ pepper, chopped

50g sliced mushrooms

25g low fat cheddar cheese, grated

Salt & Pepper to taste

Low cal cooking spray

Method:

Gently sauté the onion, mushrooms and pepper with some low calorie cooking spray. When softened, remove to a plate. Spray the pan again and pour in the beaten eggs. Gently cook the eggs for a few minutes. When the eggs starts to set, sprinkle the cheese, mushrooms, onion and pepper on top. Season with salt and pepper and fold the omelette in two to envelope the filling. Continue cooking for a further 2 mins or until the omelette is cooked through. Keep the omelette warm in an oven while you cook one for everyone else.

Pasta Carbonara

Serves: 4

Calories per serving: 315

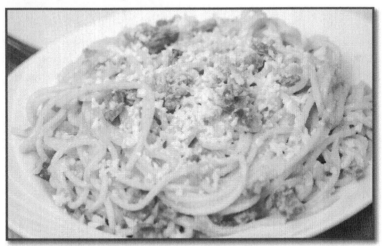

You can't go wrong with bacon, cream and pasta! Use whichever pasta you prefer; spaghetti, tagliatelle or farfalle will work really well.

Ingredients:

300g pasta

200ml low fat crème fraiche

1 free range egg

100g frozen peas

4 slices lean back bacon

20g parmesan cheese

Method:

Cook the pasta and bacon separately. When the bacon is crisp chop into small pieces. Meanwhile cook the peas (you can throw them in with the pasta for the last 6-7 minutes of cooking). Drain and put the pasta and peas back into the pan. Beat together the creme fraiche and egg and add to the pan along with the bacon. Put back on a very low heat and stir until warmed through, making sure not to turn the sauce into scrambled egg!

Sprinkle with parmesan and serve immediately.

Rustic Chicken Stew (Cacciatore)

Serves: 6

Calories per serving: 480

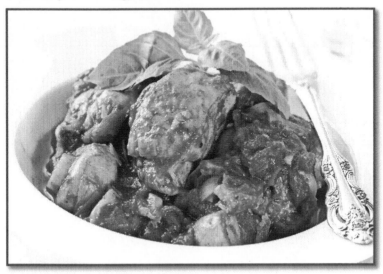

Widely known in Italy as 'Hunter's Stew'. This hearty meal has kept the faith with countless hunters and gatherers over the years. Regional variations of this dish are common throughout Italy, this rustic version is one of the most popular.

Ingredients:

1 ½ kg boned chicken pieces, skin removed

2 tbsps flour for dusting

1 onion, chopped

1 pepper, sliced

2 garlic cloves, crushed

2 400g tins chopped tomatoes

1 tsp dried rosemary

8 large pitted green olives

1 tsp anchovy paste

3 bay leaves

300ml chicken stock

Method:

Preheat the oven 160C/325F/Gas 4

Season the chicken pieces, dust with flour and then quickly brown in a large pan with a little low cal spray.

Remove the chicken from the pan and combine all the ingredients in an ovenproof dish. Bring to the boil on the stove and cover tightly. Transfer to the preheated oven for approx. 2 hours or until the chicken is cooked through and tender.

Shepherd's Pie

Serves: 4

Calories per serving 475

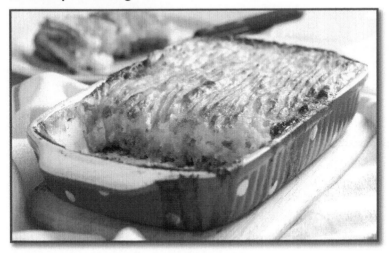

The name shepherd's pie was first recorded in the 1870's. It was originally known as *cottage pie* but people began using the term *shepherd's* when using lamb meat rather than beef which has become synonymous with cottage pie.

Ingredients:

400g lean minced lamb

1 onion, chopped

2 carrots, diced

2 stalks celery, chopped

1 garlic clove, crushed

2 tsp plain flour

50g mushrooms, sliced

1 bay leaf

1 tsp dried thyme

1 tbsp Worcestershire sauce

150ml beef stock

2 tbsp tomato purée

500g mashed potato to top the pie

Low calorie cooking spray

Method:

Preheat the oven to 180C/350F/Gas Mark 4

Brown the lamb mince in low calorie cooking spray, discarding any fat which runs off. Remove from the pan and gently sauté the onions, celery, carrots, garlic & thyme for a few minutes before stirring through the flour. Add all the other ingredients, except the mashed potato, to the pan and leave to cook for approx. 45 minutes.

Transfer the meat mixture into an oven proof dish and cover with the mashed potato. Place in the pre-heated oven for approx. 20-30 minutes or until golden and cooked through. Lovely served with peas and spring greens dressed with garlic oil.

Skinny Curry Base Mix

Makes 12 servings
Calories per serving: 37

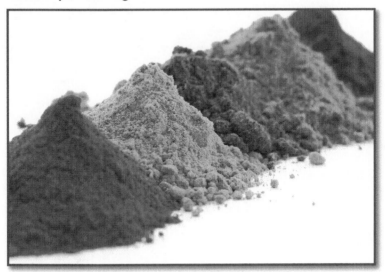

This skinny curry base sauce will form the base for both of the curries in this book. It makes sense to make up quite a big batch so you have it to hand whenever you have a curry urge.

Ingredients:

1 tbsp sunflower oil

1 large onion, chopped

2 carrots, sliced

1 tsp garlic powder

1 tsp cumin

1 tsp turmeric

1 tsp paprika

½ tsp garam masala

1 tsp ground coriander

½ tsp ground ginger

1 tsp salt

1 tsp sugar

2 tbsp tomato puree

1 400g tin chopped tomatoes

500ml chicken stock

Method:

Gently sauté the onions and carrots in the oil for a few minutes.

Add all the dried spices and tomato puree and cook for another minute or two.

Add the stock, salt, sugar and chopped tomatoes, cover and leave to simmer very gently for 40 minutes.

Blend until completely smooth then split into portions. You can chill for a few days or freeze for a few months.

Sloppy Joes

Serves: 4

Calories Per Serving 240

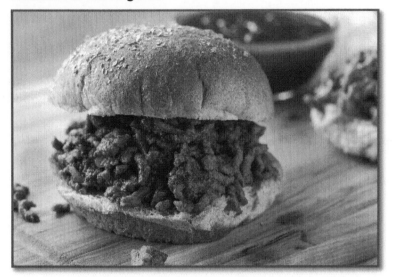

Sloppy Joes are loved by kids and adults alike. Don't worry about getting messy - the joy is in the eating not the cleaning up!

Ingredients:

450g lean ground beef

1 400g tin chopped tomatoes

1 onion, chopped

1 green pepper, chopped

1 tsp mild chilli powder

½ tsp garlic powder

½ tsp mustard powder

1 tsp soy sauce

1 tsp Worcestershire sauce

Salt & pepper to taste

Low cal cooking spray

75g ketchup or BBQ sauce

Method:

Gently brown the beef in a frying pan with some low calorie cooking spray and set to one side. In the same pan sauté the onions and pepper for a few minutes. Combine all the ingredients (except the ketchup) into the pan and cook for 30-40 mins until the beef is cooked through and the liquid has reduced. Add ketchup or BBQ sauce to your taste when serving. Lovely with toasted sandwich buns, lettuce, tomato & onion.

.

Spaghetti Bolognaise

Serves: 4

Calories per serving: 344

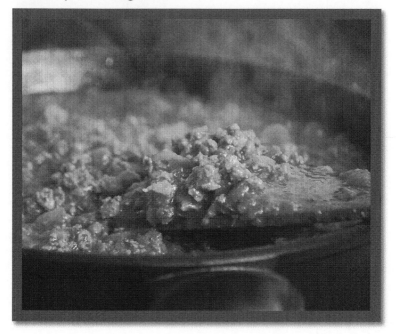

Nothing can be simpler or more satisfying than spaghetti Bolognaise. You can add mushrooms and peppers to the recipe if you like, and a dash or two of Worcestershire sauce gives extra depth.

Ingredients:

500g lean minced beef

1 400g tin chopped tomatoes

500ml tomato passata

1 tsp each dried oregano & thyme

1 stick celery, chopped

2 bay leaves

1 tbsp tomato puree

3 garlic cloves, crushed

2 onions, chopped

Low cal cooking spray

Salt and pepper to taste

Method:

Brown the meat and onions in a frying pan with a little low cal spray. Combine all the ingredients in a saucepan, bring up to heat, cover and leave to cook on low for approx. 60 minutes. Ensure the meat is fully cooked through and serve with rigatoni, penne or spaghetti. For a fuller flavour, leave to cook longer on a lower heat.

Steak Pie

Serves: 6

Calories per serving: 320

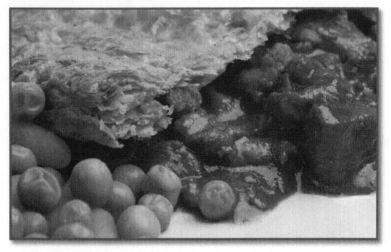

Steak pie is the heart of a great meal. You can add mushrooms to this recipe or kidney, as is traditional, if that suits your family.

Ingredients:

700g lean stewing steak, trimmed

1 onion, chopped

450ml beef stock

2 carrots, sliced

Salt & pepper to taste

2 tsp Worcestershire sauce

225g ready made low fat puff pastry

2 tsp corn flour

Splash of milk

Method:

Preheat the oven to Gas Mark 7/220°C/425°F.

Brown the steak in a pan with a little low cal cooking spray. Remove to a plate and gently fry the onion and carrots in the same pan for a few minutes. Add the meat back into the pan and add the stock, seasoning and Worcestershire sauce. Cover and leave to simmer gently for up to 2 hours, or until the meat is completely tender. Feel free to add a little water during cooking if needed. Place the cornflour in a cup and add a little water to create a paste. Add the paste to the pan and stir through to thicken.

Place the meat mixture in an ovenproof dish. Roll out the puff pastry and cover the meat. Push the edges down and trim off the sides. Brush with a little milk and bake in the pre-heated oven for 25 minutes until the pastry puffs up and is golden brown.

Sunday Roast

Serves: 4
Calories per serving: 415

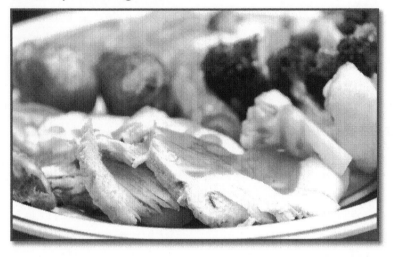

Roast dinner is still the No. 1 favourite in UK food polls. It's not just the meal that make it special, it's the idea of sitting down as a family and eating a Sunday lunch together which appeals. This is less of a recipe and more of a suggestion list, with a couple of cheat ingredients to keep the calories down.

Ingredients:

500g skinless chicken breasts (much leaner than a whole roast chicken)

350g potatoes

2 tbsp groundnut oil

2 carrots, sliced

½ head each of broccoli and cauliflower cut into floret

100g frozen peas

4 frozen yorkshire puddings

250ml Bisto style gravy

Method:

Preheat the oven to 180C/350F/Gas Mark 4

Put a roasting tin with the oil in the oven.

Peel the potatoes and cook each into 4 'roastie' size chunks. Boil in a pan of salted water for approx. 6 -8 minutes (don't let them go too soft).

Meanwhile season and very loosely, wrap the chicken breasts in tin foil. Place on a baking tray in the oven. Drain the potatoes and then add to the smoking-hot roasting tin. Brush with the hot oil and place in the top shelf of the oven.

The chicken and potatoes will need approx. 30-40 minutes or until the chicken is fully cooked and the roast potatoes are crisp and golden. Cook the vegetables while the potatoes and chicken are in the oven. A couple of minutes before you bring out the chicken, place the yorkshire puddings on the baking tray.

When it's ready, slice your chicken into carvery-style slices and arrange all the other cooked ingredients around them on the dish.

Tikka Masala

Serves 4

Calories Per Serving 402

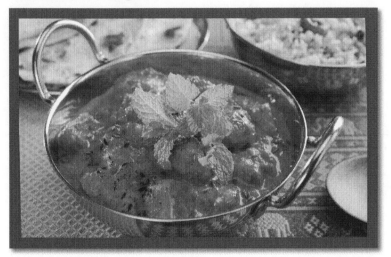

The classic British curry!

Adopted as the UK's national dish, Chicken Tikka Masala is one of the all time most popular British curries, although in recent years it has relinquished it's top dog crown to Jalfrezi.

First make the tikka

Ingredients:

600g lean meat, cubed

250ml fat free Greek yoghurt

1 tsp turmeric ground cumin, garam masala, coriander, mild chilli powder, garlic powder

½ tsp ground ginger

1 tbsp lemon juice

Pinch salt

3 drops red food colouring

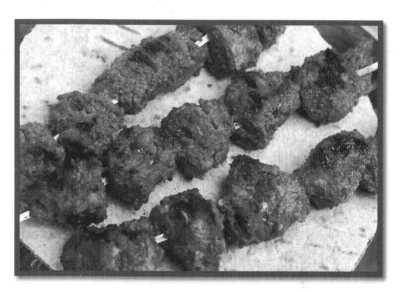

Method:

Mix all the spices, food colouring and lemon juice together to form a paste.

Add yoghurt and mix through.

Combine the meat into the mixture and leave to marinade in the fridge overnight.

Put the meat pieces on a wire rack over a baking tray and cook in a pre-heated oven at 200C/400F/Gas Mark 6 for 8-10 minutes. Turn each piece over and put back in the oven for a further 8-10 minutes or until the meat is properly cooked through.

Then use your tikka pieces to make your masala

Ingredients:

2 portions skinny curry base mix **(see page 70 for recipe)**

600g tikka pieces

1 tsp sugar

½ tsp salt

1 tsp sunflower oil

½ tsp each of garlic powder, mild chilli powder & ground ginger

1 tsp mild curry powder

4 tbsp tomato puree

4 drops natural red food colouring

4 tbsp fat free Greek yoghurt

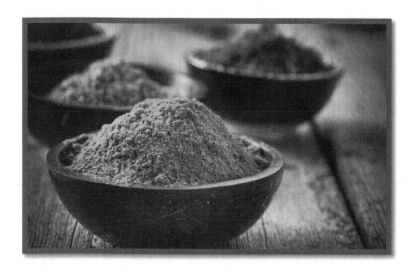

Method:

Gently warm the skinny curry base mix through in a pan.
Meanwhile heat the oil in a frying pan and add the meat tikka
pieces, ground spices & tomato puree and cook through.

Add the warmed curry base sauce, sugar and salt to the meat
mixture and stir well. Leave to heat through thoroughly until
piping hot. Take off the heat, add the yoghurt and red food
colouring to the mixture and serve straight away.

Toad In The Hole

Serves: 4

Calories per serving: 299

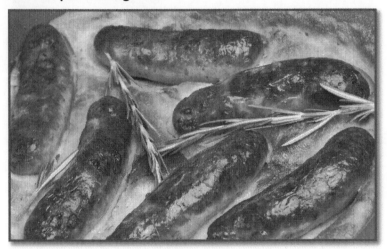

Much dispute surrounds the origin of the name of this simple dish. Some suggest the dish itself bears some resemblance to an actual toad sticking its head out of a hole but this seems unlikely! The dish is also sometimes referred to as Jimmy toad or froggy hole and is a big hit with the kids.

Ingredients:

8 thick low-fat pork sausages

1 tsp olive oil

100g plain flour

1 free range egg

300ml semi skimmed milk

2 tsp dijon mustard

½ tsp each of dried thyme and rosemary

Salt & pepper to taste

Method:

Preheat the oven to 200C/400F/Gas mark 6. Pierce the sausages, place on an oven proof dish and cook for 20 minutes in the oven.

Meanwhile make up the batter by sifting the flour into a bowl. Beat the egg into the flour and gradually add the milk, beating all the time, to create a smooth batter.

Add the dried herbs, mustard and seasoning. Cut the cooked sausages in half in the oven proof dish. Pour the batter over the top and cook in the middle of the oven for 30-40 mins or until the batter is golden brown and puffed up. Delicious with baked beans or steamed greens.

Cobb Salad

Serves: 4

Calories per serving: 446

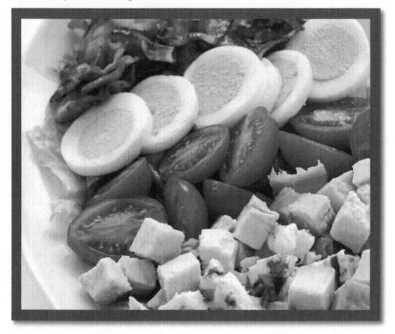

Originally created in the 1930's, Cobb Salad has become a staple for outdoor eating. There are lots of variations but the recipe here is one of the most popular.

Ingredients:

3 hard-boiled free range eggs, peeled and chopped

4 slices lean back bacon, cooked until crisp

1 head Romaine lettuce, coarsely chopped

Handful freshly chopped coriander and basil

1 Iceberg lettuce, chopped

½ cucumber, chopped

175g skinless chicken breast, cooked and cubed

2 avocados, cubed

2 tomatoes, chopped

100g blue cheese, crumbled

Dressing:

70ml extra-virgin olive oil
70ml red-wine vinegar
30g blue cheese
1 tsp Worcestershire sauce
½ tsp mild mustard
1 clove garlic, crushed
1 tsp lemon juice
¼ tsp coarse salt
½ tsp coarsely ground black pepper

Method:

Cover a plate with the chopped lettuce. On top of the lettuce arrange the ingredients into neat rows and sprinkle with the chopped coriander and basil.

For the dressing combine together the vinegar, lemon juice, Worcestershire sauce, mustard and garlic and then the blue cheese to make a paste. Add the olive oil and salt & pepper to create a thick dressing which you can pour over the prepared salad or serve on the table in a bowl for people to help themselves.

CookNation

Starters/Sides

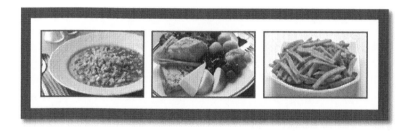

Chicken Soup

Serves: 6

Calories per serving : 188

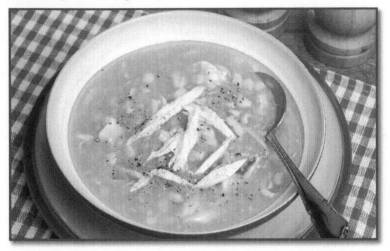

Making chicken soup couldn't be easier and you'll find it a vast improvement on most tinned varieties. You can make this smooth or chunky, whichever your family prefer.

Ingredients:

30g butter

2 onions, chopped

2 stalks celery, chopped

20g plain flour

1.2 litres chicken stock

200g cooked chicken, chopped

30g frozen sweetcorn

1 tbsp freshly chopped flat leaf parsley

Salt and pepper to season

Method:

Gently melt the butter in a pan with the onions, celery and carrots. When they begin to soften, stir in the flour and continue cooking for a few minutes. Slowly add the stock and bring the mixture up to a good simmer. Add the sweet corn and cook for approx. 10 minutes, or until everything is tender. You could at this stage puree the soup to give a smooth base before adding the chicken or, if you prefer a more hearty texture, leave as it is and throw in the chicken for a minute or two of further cooking. Season to your taste and serve with a little chopped parsley.

Cullen Skink

Serves: 4

Calories per serving: 209

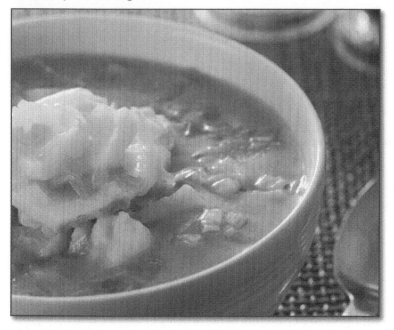

If you've never heard of Cullen Skink you might not be immediately charmed by the sound of this recipe. Think again and give it a try. Massively popular in Scotland, this potato and fish soup is fantastic.

Ingredients:

250g smoked haddock boneless fillets

1 onion, chopped

150g potatoes

300ml chicken stock

250ml skimmed milk

1 tsp low fat 'butter' spread

1tbsp low fat creme fraiche

Salt & pepper to taste

1 tbsp chopped chives

Method:

Peel the potatoes and cut into small cubes.

Melt the butter and gently fry the onions for about 3-4 minutes, add the stock and potatoes and bring up to the boil. Simmer gently for 10 minutes.

In another pan, place the haddock and milk and gently poach for 5-7 minutes until tender. Take the fish out the milk and flake into pieces. Add the fish to the potato mix along with the fishy milk and season well. Cook for another 5-10 minutes, take off the heat and add the creme fraiche. Transfer into bowl and garnish with chopped chives.

Potato Salad

Serves: 4

Calories per serving: 150

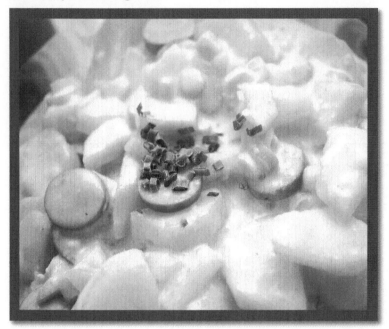

There are a million variations on potato salad. The version here is one of the most popular. Feel free to add a handful of pitted sliced olives.

Ingredients:

1 hard boiled free range egg

450g small salad potatoes

1 tbsp low fat mayonnaise

1 tbsp fat free Greek yoghurt

1 tsp extra-virgin olive oil

1 tsp dijon mustard

1 tbsp white wine vinegar

½ red pepper, chopped

2 tbsp chopped radishes

½ red onion, chopped

1 stalk celery, chopped

1 tbsp capers, chopped

2 tbsp chopped chives

Salt & pepper to taste

Method:

Cook the potatoes in salted boiling water for approx. 10-15 minutes until they are tender. Drain the potatoes and place in a bowl to cool before slicing. Meanwhile combine the mayo, yoghurt and mustard in a bowl. Add the vinegar to the potatoes and coat then gently. Combine all the ingredients together in one bowl to make the finished salad. Leave to cool and then refrigerate.

Ploughman's Lunch

Serves: 4

Calories per serving: 372

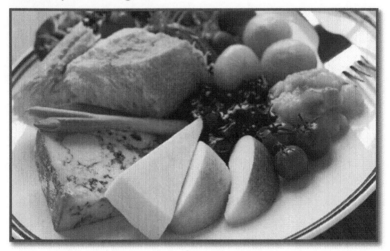

A Ploughman's lunch comes in many variations, but the classic version always contains cheese, chutney and bread. The version here is a great low fat lunch for everyone.

Ingredients:

2 apples, peeled, cored and sliced

200g low-fat cheddar cheese

100g stilton

2 Romaine lettuce heads

4 carrots, grated

1 red onion, sliced

2 slices crusty bread

Squeeze of lemon juice

4 small pickled onions

150g chutney

4 large vine tomatoes, sliced

Method:

Carefully arrange all the ingredients on 4 plates, or alternatively place everything in the middle of the table and have everyone help themselves.

Scotch Broth

Serves: 4

Calories per serving: 170

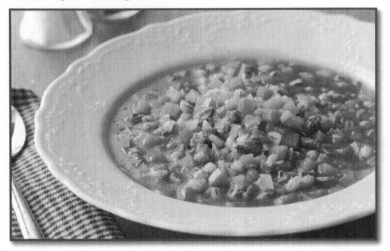

Originating from Scotland, Scotch Broth has gone on to become popular worldwide as a filling economical soup.

Ingredients:

2 onions, chopped

1 celery stalk, chopped

½ leek, sliced

50g shredded cabbage

150g pearl barley

1.8litres lamb stock

Salt and freshly ground black pepper

150g carrots, chopped

150g turnips, chopped

Method:

Place all the ingredients, except the cabbage, in a pan on a high heat. When it begins to boil, reduce the heat and leave to simmer for a minimum of 2 hours or until the pearl barley is tender. 10 minutes before the end of cooking, add the cabbage.

Sweet Potato Fries

Serves: 4

Calories per serving: 211

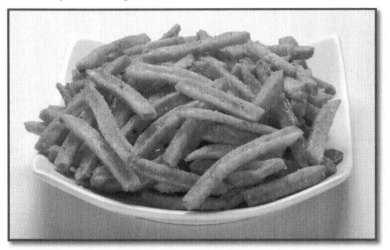

These oven baked fries are absolutely delicious and can be served both as a side dish or decadent main. Serve with ketchup and mayo!

Ingredients:

600g sweet potatoes, peeled

1 tbsp sugar

2 tsp salt

1 tsp paprika or cajun seasoning

Low calorie cooking spray

Method:

Preheat oven to 425F/220C/Gas Mark 7

Cut the potatoes in slices and then in rows to make 'fries'. You can go as thick or thin as you prefer but keep them all a similar size.

Put the raw fries into a bowl and coat with paprika, low-cal cooking spray, salt and sugar. Mix really well to make sure each is properly covered.

Spread the fries out onto a grilling rack over a baking tin. Don't pile them up, they should be a thin layer, ideally.

Bake for 20-30 minutes (depending on the thickness of your fries) or until they are crisp and brown.

CookNation

102

Desserts

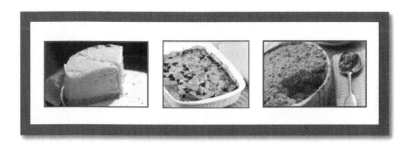

Apple Pie

Serves: 8

Calories per serving: 210

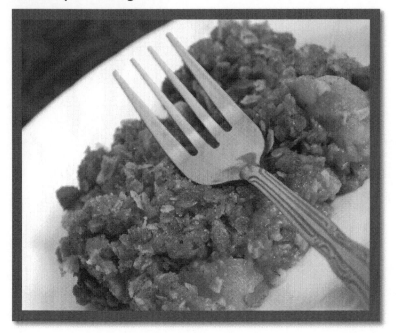

This crust-less version of apple pie makes for fewer calories but not less taste.

Ingredients:

500g cooking apples, peeled, cored and sliced

1 tsp lemon juice

1 tsp ground cinnamon

170g sugar

85g butter, melted

85g chopped pecans

1 free range egg, beaten

125g plain flour

½ tsp salt

Method:

Preheat the oven to 375F/190C/Gas Mark 5

Mix together half of the sugar with the apples, cinnamon and lemon juice.

In a separate bowl combine the butter, pecans, egg, flour, salt and the rest of the sugar. Arrange the apples in a greased 20cm tin and spread over the pecan mix. Place in a preheated oven for approx. 40-50mins or until golden brown and properly cooked through.

Blueberry Cobbler

Serves: 8

Calories per serving: 220

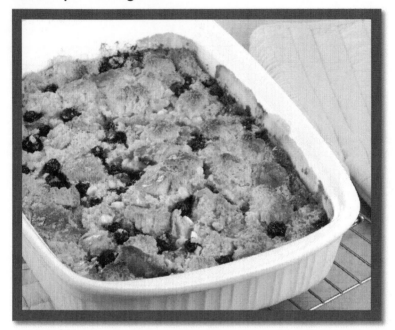

The blueberries in this recipe can be substituted for whichever is your favourite soft berry.

Ingredients:

190g plain flour

200g sugar

Pinch of salt

1 ½ tsp baking powder

175ml skimmed milk

1 tbsp butter, melted

275g blueberries

1 tsp vanilla extract

Method:

Preheat the oven to 350F/180C/Gas Mark 4

Mix together the flour, 150g of sugar, salt, and baking powder. Add the milk, butter and vanilla extract and stir well. Pour the mixture into an 8-inch baking tin. Add the fruit evenly to the pan and sprinkle with the rest of the sugar. Place in a preheated oven and cook for 40 minutes or until properly cooked through.

Bread and Butter Pudding

Serves: 4

Calories per serving: 218

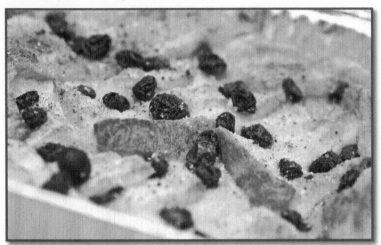

This is a bread and butter pudding without the butter. Don't worry - you won't miss it. This pudding is still delicious.

Ingredients:

8 slices bread

25g brown sugar

50g raisins

½ tsp ground nutmeg

Pinch of cinnamon

2 free range eggs

350ml semi skimmed milk

Method:

Preheat the oven to 180 C/350F/Gas Mark 4

Cut the bread slices into halves. In an ovenproof dish, arrange half the bread pieces in the base. Sprinkle with half the sugar and half the raisins, the nutmeg and cinnamon. Use the rest of the bread to make a second layer and sprinkle over the rest of the raisins. Mix together the remaining sugar, milk and eggs and gently pour over the bread. Place in the oven and leave to cook for approx. 40 minutes or until golden and cooked through.

Carrot Cake

Serves: 8

Calories per serving: 267

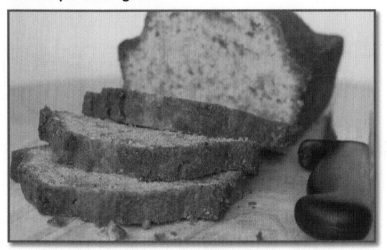

Carrot cake is a great treat for kids. It tastes fabulous and is good for you. The version here is without an iced topping, but you can add this if you like by mixing together some cream cheese and icing sugar and spreading over the top after cooking and cooling.

Ingredients:

1 tbsp poppy seeds

1 tsp baking powder

2 tsp mixed spice

¼ tsp salt

100ml sunflower oil

175g brown sugar

3 free range eggs, lightly beaten

250g grated carrots

175g wholemeal self raising flour

Method:

Preheat the oven to 180 C/350F/Gas Mark 4

Sift the flour, salt, baking powder and spice in a bowl. Make a well in the centre and add the eggs, oil and sugar. Mix well then add the carrot and poppy seeds. When everything is thoroughly combined pour into a greased 1kg loaf tin and cook for approx. 40 mins or until golden, firm to the touch and clean on the skewer test (push a wooden skewer into the cake and if it comes out clean- it's ready). Leave to cool on a wire rack and slice.

Cheesecake

Serves: 8

Calories per serving: 380

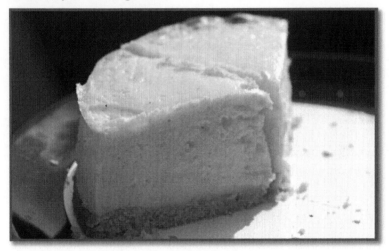

The lemon juice in this recipe give the cheesecake a light zingy zip which is lovely with ice cream.

Ingredients:

200g digestive biscuits

2 tbsp skimmed milk

450g low fat cream cheese, softened

200g sugar

1 tsp vanilla extract

3 free range eggs

200g low fat sour cream

3 tbsp lemon juice

Method:

Preheat oven to 350F/180C/Gas Mark 4

Beat together the cream cheese, lemon juice, sugar and vanilla essence and place in the fridge. Meanwhile smash the biscuits together in a plastic bag, add the milk and mix together. Press the biscuit into the base of a greased 8 inch cake tin.

Place the tin in the oven and bake for 10 minutes. Remove from oven and add the cream cheese mixture and bake for a further 20 minutes or until the cheesecake mixture is cooked through. Leave to cool and place in the fridge to firm up before slicing and serving.

Pancakes

Serves: 4

Calories per serving: 160

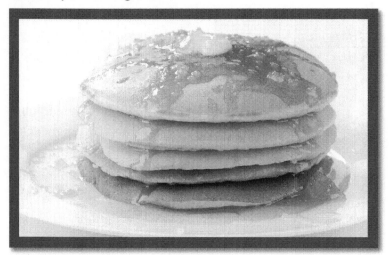

These pancakes are lovely just as they are but even better with fresh blueberries.

Ingredients:

125g plain flour

1 tsp baking powder

½ tsp salt

2 tbsp caster sugar

120ml milk

1 free range egg, lightly beaten

2 tbsp olive oil

Handful of fresh blueberries (optional)

Method:

Sift together the flour, baking powder, salt and caster sugar. Separately mix together the milk, egg and olive oil. Beat the egg mixture into the flour mixture thoroughly. Add the blueberries and leave to stand for a few minutes

Heat up a dry non-stick frying pan. When the pan is hot, partially fill a ladle with pancake mixture and pour into the pan. Cook until it begins to bubble then flip over for a further minute. Remove to a plate in a warmed oven and keep on going until all the pancake mixture is finished. Delicious with maple syrup.

Rhubarb Crumble

Serves: 4

Calories per serving: 282

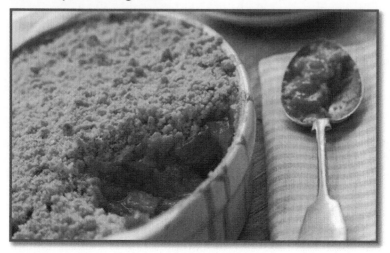

Generally thought of as a fruit, rhubarb is in fact a vegetable which is delicious in this 'fruit' crumble.

Ingredients:

120g plain flour

50g butter, cubed

450g stewed rhubarb (make this by 'stewing' chopped rhubarb in a pan for 20mins with a tbsp each of sugar and water)

3 tbsps water

1 tsp ground cinnamon

1 tsp ground nutmeg

10g brown sugar

Method:

Preheat the oven to 350F/180 C/Gas Mark 4

The quickest way to make the crumble is to place the cubed butter and flour into a food processor and gently pulse until it turns into crumbs. Make sure you don't over pulse it though as it will stick together. Spoon the stewed rhubarb into a small oven proof dish then sprinkle with the nutmeg and cinnamon. Cover with the crumble mixture and sprinkle with sugar. Place in the oven and cook for approx. 30-40 minutes or until it's golden brown and cooked through.

Rice Pudding

Serves: 4

Calories per serving: 170

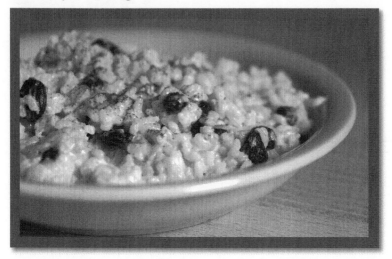

Rice pudding is a dish enjoyed by the people of almost every continent of the world. This European version was exported to the US by immigrants in the latter part of the 20th century.

Ingredients:

100g pudding rice

½ tsp ground cinnamon

50g brown sugar

85g raisins or sultanas

700ml skimmed milk

pinch ground nutmeg

1 bay leaf

Large knob of unsalted butter

Method:

Pre heat the oven to 180C/350F/Gas Mark 4.

Add the rice, sugar, butter, milk and bay leaf to an oven proof dish and place in the oven for 40-50 minutes, or until the rice is tender and the milk absorbed. Sprinkle over the nutmeg before serving and remove the bay leaf. Lovely served with a dollop of jam.

You May Also Enjoy Other CookNation Titles

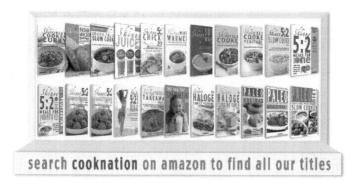

search cooknation on amazon to find all our titles

If you enjoyed *The Skinny 5:2 Family Favourites Recipe Book* we'd really appreciate your feedback. Reviews help others decide if this is the right book for them. Thank you.

You may also be interested in other titles in the CookNation series. Search 'CookNation' under Amazon.